KNOWN

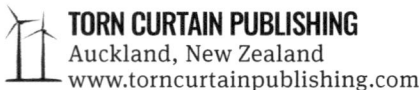

TORN CURTAIN PUBLISHING
Auckland, New Zealand
www.torncurtainpublishing.com

ISBN Softcover 978-1-991299-21-5
ISBN EPub 978-1-991299-22-2

Typeset in Georgia, Myriad Pro and Anaktoria

Cataloguing in Publishing Data
  Title: Known
  Author: Heather Pound
  Subjects: Poetry, Inspiration, Healing, Personal growth, Mental health, Nature, Spirituality, Christian faith and living.

A copy of this title is held at the National Library of New Zealand.

KNOWN

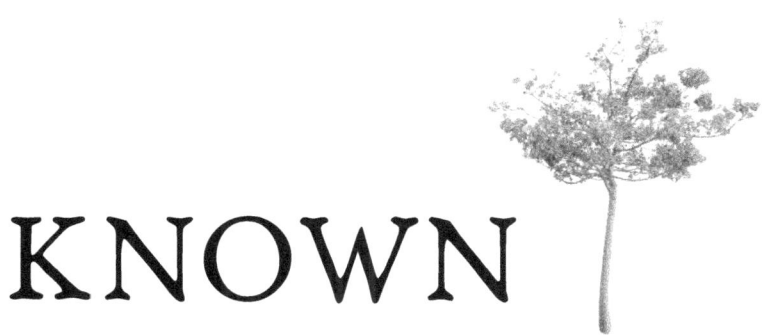

Poems of perspective and growth

HEATHER POUND

i do not wish for you
wealth, success or fame
but that you might live your life
one savored moment at a time.
that you might put your hand
to something worthwhile
discover satisfaction in giving
and that your days brim full
with chosen community
creativity . . . and Light.

— dedicated to the four precious souls
that call me 'mom'.

Contents

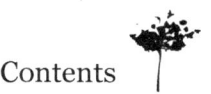

Introduction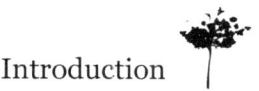

Writing has always been a way to know myself, to understand what might be hiding beneath the noise in my head and figuring out what my heart is really saying. If anything really good or really hard happened, it went down on a page.

One day I sat, journal in hand, seeking to process something historical that had raised its head and was impacting me that day. Because it was so deep and integral, however, the words just wouldn't flow. It came out in bits and pieces, chopped back, that began to form prose on the page. I remembered then how I loved to write poetry in my teens, and a new and improved way of processing my thoughts was born.

There's something about this way of writing, the seeking of the exact right words, the layout for emphasis, the getting rid of the dross and only saving the best, that is—for me, at least—a fantastic way to work with thoughts and to better know myself. It also fuels my creative part and in return makes me a better observer of humanity and beauty.

These poems were written over several years and were chosen from pages that included many more. Since I am a counsellor, there is a strong theme of mental wellbeing, but also thoughts around relationships, motherhood, nature, beauty, faith, light and hope. It is my wish that they also model perspective and maybe even stimulate a bit of growth. They certainly have in me.

The need to know ourselves, our thoughts, values, passions, what brings us joy and what makes us 'tick', is part of being human. So is the desire to deeply know others and the world around us—and in return, to be authentically, powerfully KNOWN. Here's to the journey of life!

Let's keep inviting each other along for the ride.

today i choose to gather
dewy-fresh, not yet dried by the sun
soft green stems, unaffected by wind
bits and pieces present, but often brushed aside unnoticed.

i will gather joy, not because it is scarce, but because without it
how is a life to be lived?
it is the food that sustains us, yet we try to survive
with stolen morsels, a guilty pleasure
quickly consumed lest someone else notice,
then back to more important things at hand.

but what is a life without joy?
grasp it by the face and kiss its mouth.
it is companionship not only sweet but
necessary to ease the cracks in our souls,
to soften calloused flesh within.

i will gather joy now while it may be found
like jewels layered beneath thick autumn leaves,
not really hidden, yet inconspicuous, unseen
until you pay attention and catch the glimmer
where the sun breaks through the trees and shines,
and bending down you rustle and grasp that which sparkles
to put it in your pocket.

    — let the gathering of joy become a habit.

when you have so much to do, take a moment and just *be*.
the list will still be there, but your peace might not.

stop. feel the warmth of the sun. listen to the twitter of the bird.
really look out the window, just stare.
touch the texture of the fabric, breathe in the crisp autumn air.
taste the crème of your coffee, feel your feet on the floor.
the order doesn't matter, the specifics just a random suggestion.
simply notice,
engage your senses.

then, just be present . . .

. . . for at least a few hundred beats of your heart.
breathe in, breathe out, and be.

this is the vital thing, what connects you to yourself.
give the brain a chance to quiet the worry and whisper what is best.
give your heart a chance to feel, tense muscles relax
physiology working in harmony.

teach your body to remember this space
this necessary dialling down
honouring the container that serves you,
the soul that feeds you.
listen to what it wants to tell you.

— if we don't listen, our body finds ways to tell us anyway.

these bodies that i birthed into existence
precious like no other.
growing, changing, spreading their wings.
i want them to fly, but still . . .

these hours that we linger in the same space
laughing, talking, just simply being
these are the moments worth savouring.

i drink in all that they are, filing away snapshots and smiles.
mental pictures to pull out later and savour
a steaming cup of cocoa on a brisk winter's night,
nourishing warmth to my soul.

bittersweet memories of giggles and tiny toes
now walking slower, more measured, grown.
soft cheek became angled jaw, yet none the less adored
a masterpiece of heart and womb.

fly, little bird, fly
but remember you can come back to rest.
i've sheltered you from the storm before, i can do it again.
spread your wings, grow stronger, but always know
there's a safe space for you in my arms.

we know the taste of sweet
because of bitter
of joy because of pain
of peace because of turmoil.
this enormous sense of
treasure held deep within
because we also know of loss.

one really does not exist
without the other.

this does not make the
painful portions easier
to bear, but it does invite us
to value, to notice
and to relish the good
and by default be more
accepting of the rest.

when painful comes to call
consider this. and when the
world is full of sunshine and
smiles, soak that in as well.
gather from each day what
is given, and you will find
more balance in the end.

no matter what your thoughts tell you
on this particular morning fresh,
no matter what life has thrown your way
in challenges and in highs and lows,
there is always possibility.

do not think that joy has passed you by
like a tornado jumping house to house,
striking one and missing yours, never catching you up
in her tremendous grasp.

because perhaps for you she will come as the
gentlest scent on a summer breeze, pregnant
with humidity and not necessarily familiar
or comfortable.

all i know is that joy is not stingy, she does
not snub or distinctions make. no, she is
a friend to each and every one willing
to draw her in.

if she has not recently your way come,
then make sure you allow
yourself to linger in the kinds of spaces
she might frequent.

because sooner or later, she will arrive,
freshly bathed and dressed in her best,
and you must be ready to welcome her
in friendship and cheerful conversation

or even in peaceful quiet and flickering
firelight. just enjoy her presence
and her careful, ministering manner.

— lean in, lean in to joy's gaze.

i have always known that 'his yoke is easy, his burden light'
but i used to think of him holding the reins, myself the ox-calf,
him a loving master, tending my wounds and needs
directing my steps, choosing what is best
while *my* neck carried the harness.

it's important to remember though, that a yoke has more space.
not one, but places for two necks and two shoulders
binding two creatures together in helpful companionship.
moving in the same direction, following the same commands
bearing the burden, doing the work, feeling the chafe
—together.

this God that i know is of the sort that doesn't leave me to
walk the field of life alone. he is not remote, out of reach
or jostling from behind.
no, he dips his neck, accepts the yoke
and walks beside

sharing my burden,
feeling the dust and the sun and the thirst.
he willingly supports and offers strength
for both the pleasant and the pain.

the yoke is easy and the burden is light
because *he* shoulders the heaviest load.

— when you think you're alone and God doesn't care.

luxuriously she stretches, the cat lying in the sun
as if to say, this
this is the way to start the day
and to pause often after.

the sun's rays will come again, of course
but this one, this sunbeam that has 150 million kilometres come
only to shine this minute
will be gone.

i used to think that papaya
tasted like cheap perfume
until while living in the islands
a papaya tree sprang up right outside my door.

the freshness must intensify
the goodness, i reckon.
flesh still warm from the sun, juice dripping
scraping away multitudes of black seed balls
before scooping out the sustenance.

i learned to drop those seeds straight into the rubbish
because that same tree taught me
that for a plant that springs tall fast
appealing and willowy in the wind
the roots that lie beneath the surface
are ruthless

because one day very little water
came from the tap and when we found
the culprit
—it was that jolly pawpaw tree.

tempting us with fruit
but roots spreading rapidly, puncturing pipes.
the plumber that knew about these things
said you cannot let one spring up
right against the house.
the damage that comes is swift
unexpected and surprisingly fierce.

so, you must pull out those tree sprouts
for quite a few steps away from your walls
protect the boundary, the important
from the tyranny of something
that looks sweet in the moment
but wrecks the supply of something vital.

in the terrible night of the soul
when your senses only find storm
you long to dull, block out the pain
roll into fetal—protect.

but even though it hurts
more than you think you can bear,
if you open your eyes sufficient to squint
take hands from your ears every now and again
—you might be amazed

because pain, the offender
does not journey alone.

he arrives with gems,
lucky finds that wait to be gathered.
jewels that grasp on to coattails fierce
and say things like 'there is always hope.'

they rejuvenate
like a cup of cold water in parched locales
offering gifts like healing
and 'life might be worth living'
and kindness.

if you clasp them in your hands
to keep your ears uncovered
you might begin to hear the song
beneath the surface, but louder grows.

the music of dreams and longings
and the hope of beautiful things
that feed your soul in the darkness
instructing you in the deeper things of life

until the arrival of dawn.

you can do your utmost to persuade me
of all the world's ills
but this, my friend, you need not do.

for I have seen with my own two eyes
depravity
malice and greed.

i have heard with my own two ears
the cries of beatings
the keening wails of grief, of bondage, of hope defiled.

i have held the hands that death will visit soon
and seen children as shadows begging for bread
granted apathy in return.

i have attentively observed over time what human beings
are capable of
and i lament.

i am still . . .

but then

the song awakens in my chest
softly first but louder grows
and no matter what i have seen and heard or felt with my frame
music bursts forth from my soul once again—alive

and from my lips an ancient song.
and with the hope of a thousand generations past
and of children yet to come, i cry

there is light, there is light, there is light
and this, no darkness can steal.

call me a dreamer or call me a fool
this will always be my song.

if choice looms before you in a way that overwhelms
too many options, too little time, a surplus of possible outcomes
the opinions of others always too present

if you don't know what to do, it might just be okay
to choose the one that brings *you* peace
and encourages the wholeness and wellbeing
of your very own heart

> — don't automatically choose the hardest path
> just because you 'should'.

when the workmen dug beside the road
nine months ago or more
the digger damaged branches on the tree
that has lived far longer
than i have been alive

and now that the sun warms
and new life trims the bare
with green leaves of lace unspoiled,
the gash in her new season dress
is once again—obvious.

while otherwise tall and graceful
she dances in the wind.
the broken branches naked, unmoving
remind me of a limp.

and i wonder—
do you walk with a limp like this old sister fair?
do you see the glaring wound
more than the beauty of the whole,
wish it were gone, will it away
and discover this an impossible task?

some of us walk with an unseen limp, a part of who we are.
at times it's more obvious than others
but regularly it reminds us
to stride more measured, pacing ourselves
for the journey ahead, not just a single event.

and this, while irritating, can invite us to notice
things we would have otherwise rushed on past.
worthwhile, kind, and beautiful things
there to be gathered. colourful blossoms waiting
beside the path.

and while we may resist this process
the best way forward is—acceptance

embracing all the parts of who we are
moving forward as a whole
cherishing the whole

      — even the limp.

in that vulnerable time before sleep
depression and loneliness and things like
these might come to call
—but do not allow them to wail too loud
or cause a mighty roar.

they might simply be linked to *tired*.
so, notice them, yes. say 'i see you there, welcome'
then let them be what they are
accept them, and rest.

if they visit again, then you may listen.
they do not come to depress, but to offer useful information
of what your heart might be trying to speak
but your brain hasn't acknowledged yet.

these feelings are not fatal
but clues to instruct, things that you
need to know to intentionally bring
balance, adjustment, change
and wellness to your soul.

— let the feelings teach you.

tonight i cooked a pumpkin,
one of those planted in the ditch of his retirement village
a few months back
a twinkle in his eye when he told us.
contraband in placement
collaboration with the man that cuts the grass.

i curried it and fed it to his son, my husband.
the one that looks like him
and carries his form in character.
a man of high standards for himself and a heart that gives
—but a *character* all the same when that twinkle in the eye
unanticipated comes.

'just give it a go' he told his kids, and they did
achieving much in life in the ways that make meaning—and joy
lavishness in legacy.

a lot can happen in a few short months:
the gardener now sleeps,
someone else harvests the crops
but the many things that he grew
live on

hold onto hope for someone you love.
keep it safe, lock it up tight.

when their world isn't turning
or their off-tilt axis spinning
this is the gift you can give.

hold it with care, safe
do this for them until
they find it themselves
once more.

— there is always, always hope.

the blackbird chirping outside knows
that his song while fine
will never be the nightingale

still he lifts his melody
to dusk and daybreak
full-voiced, impassioned, free.

humans, however, tend to compare
and wither in the doing.

why don't we, like the blackbird
gaze upon the dawn instead?

and remember there is enough beauty
for us all to participate and that
our own unique presentation
is exquisite and worthy and fine.

> — don't compare your gifts with others,
> simply bring your own.

you went outside into nature to ponder
and found you were sitting on empty,
scooped out like watermelon rind
flesh devoured on a hot summer day
and discarded in the sun.

then fear began to whisper tight and cruel
that you would not have what it takes
for the next wave that life might bring
or even the very next day.

fear mushroomed, sucked your breath
and wailed 'meaningless, empty, fruitless
and useless'.

words like these are quicksand to the human heart
if any attention is given.

but then you remembered
that a vessel that is empty can always catch the rain
simply by embracing its shape—hollow.

and instead of a place of lack
empty became a container to be filled
and you looked beyond yourself and saw
all the wondrous things about,
waiting to be chosen.

> — 'empty' is not a destination, it is the beginning of
> being filled with something new.

the next chair over sits a man
strong, resilient, kind—and just
a little bit tough to the outside world.
but on his arm rests a bundle
soft and furry and feline
trusting, enjoying
his companion.

every once in a while, a pat
not conscious, just being together.
a window into the softness
not everyone sees.

kindness, yes, but tenderness is the gift
he gives only to those he lets near
those closest to his heart

but animals see right into the container
to the playful gentleness within
and offer their devotion.

kind of like this poet
who should be getting ready for her day
but was moved to stop and notice.

i want to remind you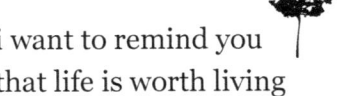
that life is worth living

that while unknown and scary it seems
while locked up away in your safe place

there is more right outside the door
than the things that caused the retreat

that living is a muscle
that must be stretched and built
through consistency and practice and time

but if you look back later
after even a small bit of exercise
you will see that you have grown

that you are stronger than before
that you are safe

so, please take a risk
even if you have already tried
time and time again

please do it once more
and open that door

when i lived in the desert, i had no respect for cacti
they were everywhere, prickly, even dangerous
if you fell into them whilst catching a ball
this my son knows well

i longed for green, famished—
soft grass, tall trees, *anything* different than these

but now i dwell where there are shades of green
more hues than even imagined before
enough to daily stop and stare
i relish this

but wouldn't you know
the houseplants i now adore
are those same spiny things i couldn't wait
to move away from

made precious by the simple fact
that they can be admired one by one
individuals, different,
monuments to creativity and protection—and beauty
i faithfully nurture these and rejoice when they respond

this causes me to question why we worry
when we're perceived *different*
because different is rare, treasured even
and rare is beautiful

—this a diamond knows well.

find a cosy spot and sit calm
and still—and notice
what is the thing that you would most
like to discover living in the innermost
part of your chest?
then put aside ridiculous distractions
keeping you apart

—and do all that it takes to find it.

i do not need to put on my best dress
wash my face or even change my attitude
in order to come to you

i do not need to clear my jumbled mind
or speak coherently
—you just say 'come'

the invitation is there and free
and all i need to do
is to bring
me

there was a time when trauma roared
vibrations under skin, constant.
inappropriately it escalated whenever it chose.

electrified brain, galloping heart, splintered vision
at odds with thought
and despotically, cold-heartedly
—inconvenient.

the most basic parts of our brains get confused
the off-and-on switch
stuck tiresomely in between.
trying to help, but just
—dysregulated.

the fortunate ones will one day
speak of such things
gloriously in past tense.

this does not mean that sounds do not startle
adrenaline releases too easily
but increasingly more pliant, manageable
more often than not.

it is as if one day after the sacred
demanding work that is healing,
we choose to climb out of cocoon, released
look up at the sky
        unfurl soft wings
                and say . . .

"this space i've been in, it no longer fits.
i need to move about, wobble away.

although this has been my story
will always be my story
my life is now bigger than this."

— there is hope within the cocoon of trauma and ptsd.

when you feel heavy or tired and you don't know why
it could be that your heart is singing of loss
and begging you to listen.

loss isn't always obvious and shouldn't be compared
to how others may have it worse
or how it is better than it used to be.

loss, is loss, is loss
it just is.

so, if your heart is trying to tell you
about something such as this
—listen
then say its name.

it may be as simple as a loss of connection, or a relationship
or loss of a freedom
even though everything else *should* be fine.

if we don't pay attention when asked
that loss swirls—and expands
and bigger and louder becomes

it screams
until we are covered by storm-clouds
dense and dark and threatening.

but if we just take time to notice the loss
and give it a name—it will breathe,
help the heart and brain consider the grief together.

and soon something that seemed so huge
and swirling, scary and loud
becomes more manageable.

so much so that it might even fit
between your two strong hands.

a plump little song thrush
perched on top of the apple tree
where dewy leaves appeared only just this week

it sat nonchalant as if to say,
'no need to look. i am just watching the day pass by'
but the worm waving in its beak when its head flicked back and
forth
told a somewhat different tale.

the charade continued until other birds in the garden flitted away
and seagulls overhead soared past, wings outstretched wide.
then purpose, intentionally hidden, struck sudden and sure.

leaping into the air, an arrow towards a target
the thrush shot into the hedge

hopefully high enough that my inquisitive cat
will not find the babies most certainly nestled there.

— things are not always what they seem.

today is blustery, miserable and damp.
one of those spring days that you must endure
for all the glorious ones that will come.

but as the wind screams fierce at my window
two little quail peck happily in my garden
fat and fluffy, plumes on top cheerfully dancing as if to say
(while i watch in stillness from porthole above)

'you can praise the strong wind for our choice of shelter
we relish this break that your hedge provides
and this soggy turf is ideal in the search for worms.'

so, as the wind continues to howl
i nod back in cheerful realisation that
if it wasn't for the less-than-perfect day

i would have missed seeing something
perfectly beautiful indeed.

     — there are treasures worth noticing
     in the midst of imperfect.

when we walked through the rose garden
and you noticed the droplets of dew on petals of cream
that had seen better days

this is the moment i knew
—you would be okay.

because a person that can see the beauty in moments like these
has the skills required to gather the light one ray at a time
and to broaden the cracks to let more sunshine in.

be a seeker of the Light.
grow this habit
hold it tight
look for the small and insignificant things
that are beauty at its core

and you will always have the perspective
needed to lift your eyes from your own despair
on those awful and terrible days that come as a part of life
and to notice something beautiful in the world once again.

and then to remember that you, yes you
are also a part of this.

> — this is your one job today: look for something,
> anything beautiful.

once i saw a lady laughing with her friends
and instinctively whispered
"if i was like her, i would always be confident"
of this i was immediately certain.

with photos reviewed, i was however surprised.
this face would not launch a thousand ships
and her figure was softer—like mine

and i pondered this for a while
and realised
it was in her smile.

for when eyes twinkled and teeth said hello
a veil lifted, and for that moment you viewed
the glorious garden inside
fully blossomed, fragrant, and free.

and this woman—she *smiled*.

she was a gardener who tended what mattered
flowers bloomed, vines encircled
accepting both sunshine and rain

and then bravely, often, and when she chose
she waived the admission fee.

she was beautiful
and i wonder still if she even knows?

open your heart, my love, to the possibility
that hope might burst forth again
that even though the journey is long
and the current path is full of thorns and stones
and bandits that steal

and even if you are convinced that nothing
in this big broad world will ever change—at least for you
that perhaps it will

perhaps it will
and perhaps your future will hold
all the things that you ever wanted

and even though today the meal served is crumbs
they are enough to sustain
for now

and even if your eyes are dry because all your tears are shed
you just might smile again

you see it there
the glimmer on the horizon, nought but a speck at first

this is proof that hope does exist
and that you still have the vision to see
that glorious change is possible

open your eyes once again to see
it may be far-far in the distance
but you need not be dismayed

take a breath in slow, and remember
that there is always something ahead to look forward to

—open your heart to see.

now is the time—do not delay
this is the day for something new

for freedom to begin
for the life that you live
to become the one that you choose.

focus on the depths to discern
what keeps your heart stagnant
what is this saying,
why is this here?

now is the time to address things like fear
to stare down its eyes, bloodshot red
—it does not know more than you
cannot the future see
no matter what it claims

all it will do is hijack your now
stealing precious energy and time
that is better spent with thoughts
that will encourage and expand

now is the time to not be afraid of sad
let it rear its longing mouth up to the air
to breathe

sadness is the lack of something precious
so give it the air it needs
to say what it needs to say
feel what it needs to feel

for it would prefer to trundle off
to the place of healing rather than sit
cold and alone in the dark
its intentions not evil, but good

now is the time to stare down the giants that have
blocked your path for far-far too long
now is the time to see them for what they are

—now is the time to fight.

what will you do when love comes to call
knocking on the door of your sombre heart

are you comfortable
too comfortable
in the place that you have been
or will you open the sash up wide
to let love's sunshine in

it's really up to you
you get to choose

pay attention to your heart when the cobwebs come
what little spiders have busily begun their webs
name them by name—then invite them to leave
because you have something else you would rather
design there instead

you may have been living the only way you know how
but if you open your heart to new ways of being
of living
of doing
you might be surprised by what is already
waiting at your door impatient

what would it be like to invite love in?

would you sit by the fire
socks on
coffee in hand

or would you kick off your shoes
and together dance?

once again you get to choose
no one will make you do this

there is a lot in this world well beyond your control
but not this
this is yours
this is your gift

do you ever look in the mirror and wonder,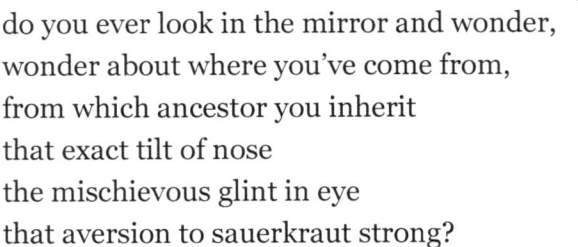
wonder about where you've come from,
from which ancestor you inherit
that exact tilt of nose
the mischievous glint in eye
that aversion to sauerkraut strong?

a tapestry of possibilities
that narrowed down,
      down,
down
to become *you*

there might be nothing new under the sun
in general
but there has never before been this exact
combination

the way you walk and talk
your particular set of talents—or weaknesses
your formative history, relationships that
have influenced

lifelong stories collected that dance around
and intertwine as your opinions form
what makes you laugh or smile,
what interests hold your mind

there has never before been
and will never ever be again—
a more you version of you

please recognise that you, my friend
are one of a kind, the rarest of rare
an undeniable original signed

take yourself out into the world
and treat yourself with all the
respect, tenderness and care
that you require

—and remember to appreciate the details
of other masterpieces too.

it has taken quite a few years, but i think i am now close to
seeing myself the way that you have *always* seen me

competent, kind, talented, even a little bit wise
—and equal, especially this.
something i had never really been offered before.

you chose a partner, someone to share life with
but also, to discuss deep topics, and to make decisions
—together.

this, the precious gift you presented on the day we wed
but something i did not dare to dream
you actually meant for quite a few years.
my history, my culture, myself, always in the way

but you have made me believe
that i have the freedom to do significant things
and have the abilities required as well
and you are happy—nay, jubilant—to cheer me on.

and would you believe that i, who can usually say
just what i want when it comes to thoughts on a page
struggle to put into words just how much this means,
how much *you* mean to this heart set free.

and how deeply and ardently i appreciate
the gift of being yours, this healing
and for the relationship that we now have
but that you always intended
—as partners.

roll down the windows of life
and let the sun stream in.
who cares if wind tangles your hair
or makes eyes water even.

live your life, experience it, cherish the day
chase meaning and purpose absolutely
—but do not forget to also have fun

live your life as a series of todays
one moment of focus at a time
gather close all of the produce that
your tended garden-of-choice has to offer

for there is beauty breath-taking
belly-laughter, moments of peace
and love beyond understanding

this is the offering, the feast available
the nourishment for a soul
who desires to live well

if you have survived on crumbs
for far, far too long
then muster all of your courage

and roll down the windows wide

i live in that bewildering place 'in-between'
not knowing when i need people—or when i just need me

(stage 1)
from chrysalis, safe and warm, slips out one wing ready to fly.
but wait, i'm not quite ready, i need a bit more time.
wing back in, relieved.
alone is great
hiatus is healing
peace.

(stage 2)
fear. of. missing. out.
they did that without me, really?
i *so* would have gone
spread my wings with joy, dancing.
people are the best, they're what i need.
this pupa thing is lonely
constricting, claustrophobic—let. me. out.

(stage 3)
i say *yes*. it's amazing
slipping off to sleep smiling, pondering the next exciting thing
making plans with my people, thinking about meeting new ones.
why didn't i do this sooner, know that this is what i need?
lingering over laughter, the topics run deep
the feast is plentiful, the talk satisfying,
a bountiful, beneficial banquet.
togetherness is best

—my wings frantically fluttering with freedom
begin to
wither.

(stage 4)
this morning i just can't fly
i can't do people, they exhaust me.
spent.
i grab my cocoon and slip back in.
it fits just right
nurturing.
why did I ever leave?

— sometimes introverted and sometimes extroverted.

it matters not if i agree
with your thoughts
or to which side
of a debate you might
attune your ear

if your words when you
speak are full of snark
if you mock your fellow man
and seem to forget

that they too, are
made in *The Image*
then my own ears
tend to narrow and
i struggle to hear
you speak.

(perhaps that is a weakness of my own)

your attitude
reflects your heart
and invites me to wonder
what character may dwell inside

and what motives you may possess
—for at the very least
as human beings, we can choose
courtesy towards our fellow man
even if and especially when . . . we disagree.

for how else will we ever
come to appreciate
that other opinions
might enhance
or clarify our own
and that, regardless
we are all human—together?

overcast but pleasant, gentle salty breeze
good company, coffee cup in hand
we watched six serious older men
running a regatta of remote-controlled sails
one metre high
and two small boys 'surfing' on water
without waves, laughing free—
and although i have seen much to challenge
this before, any doubts i may have fostered
that humanity still has something good left to offer
sailed off with the breeze.

today

look at someone you love
and say:

"you don't need
to do a thing
or be a thing
or achieve
any single thing
to be valued—
you just are."

repeat it again to some people
that mean the world
from a heart that truly
believes it for those
that you adore.

then look in the mirror
and say it again—
for that is also true.

all those niggling worries and deeply felt fears
that you have carried for far, far too long
have mostly come to naught,
i remind you gently of this

there are things in your grasp
and things that are not
and most of your worries
fall into the latter

you are strong but it is okay
to lay these things down,
the weight of the world entire
is just too much to bear

so let it go
be free
take back only
what bears your name

hold these up to the Light
and wisdom for them seek

but all the rest—they will tear you down
squash you into something small
shatter your wellbeing

i wish i had known this aeons ago
but you are a single cup
just a small thing really
and all you need to do

is to keep your cup filled
running over, even

this cup that is you
is all you need to be
and worry has no place
within your porcelain frame

when you don't know where you're going
or even what you're doing
—just take one step.

when your chest won't stop constricting
and the air's unfit for breathing
—just take one breath.

when movement is exhausting and
your feeble limbs are freezing
—just make one movement more.

when clouds obscure your vision and
you can't see the horizon
—just fly one moment more.

just take one step, breathe one breath
make one movement, fly one moment
—or sometimes just exist.

later you will look back on the road once traveled
and discover that you made it
through unbearable fire
through piercing cold
through labyrinths where senses failed

that you fought a mighty battle
and were unexpectedly triumphant
—one step, one breath, one movement
and one moment at a time.

you know what it's like to watch the pain of someone you love
wishing with your entire heart and soul that you could
with your own two hands reach into every crevice
each cell and atom of their body—and heal.

but alas, while humans can do many amazing things
we cannot accomplish this.

you are not here to give any well-meaning
planned out words of wisdom, platitudes of hope.
these your loved one has already encountered enough.

you are here to listen to whatever needs
to escape their worn-out, tattered heart
and to offer a safe and quiet space
—for rest.

if they wonder how you have managed to
keep on breathing in circumstances such as these
you can happily offer whatever thoughts you have
—but only if they ask.

until then, just *be*.

> — presence is a powerful gift, simply offer this.

God and i had a conversation
that felt a little one-sided
where i went on and on
about all of the things
i needed him to fix
and change

or at least help me
to feel better about
or understand even

i asked him why he was
moving so slow

why things had happened
in the first place

and where he was at the time
anyway.

when my thoughts came to an end
breathless, and i turned at last
to meet his gaze

i wondered how a face could
weep with sorrow and be so
full of love and peaceful joy
at the very same time

and all he replied was
"i hear you, just trust me

if this has not turned into
something beautiful or good
then i have not finished yet."

—hold on to the light

you must
(notice this please—i did not say *should* but *must*)
you must offer understanding to all of the versions of you
all the various *yous* that you recall

stop holding them to the standard
that you expect today
judging them with older and wiser eyes

blaming them for what they did and did not do
the places they failed or caused you pain
when they were only young

instead, be the kindest of kind
offer them a seat on the sofa comfy,
pillow plumped behind back
feet raised
hot cocoa cup in hand

thank them one by one for all the adventures
the journeys you have taken together, and the things
they practiced long and taught

perhaps you will be inspired again
by their youthful flair
by feet that used to twirl
costume sorted, audience or not

celebrate their innocence and the naivete
that allowed them to believe the best
of everyone they met

you have things to learn from them
they have wisdom too

be especially kind to the mother of children young
doing the best that she knew how with no knowledge
of roads and curves that lay ahead

offer tenderness to the version that hurt
that absorbed and held much pain
she did this to allow the rest of you
to function, to carry on

this one, that one
and all the ones in-between
they are important
they matter
they have led to who you are

— one and all, they are welcome here and loved

i wonder what it will take
to rewrite the story
you hear inside your mind?

as you speak:
you hear victim
i hear survivor.

you see failure
i see endurance.

you smell fear
i catch the scent
of courage.

you touch the tears
on your face with shame
and apologise.

i understand how your
heart needs release and
how weeping is a sign of
someone brave enough
to recall and speak of painful things.

words create stories, and my hope
is that by re-weaving consonants
and vowels you will rewrite yours in
your own unique way and in your
personal time into something similar
to what i and others . . . already see.

please don't run from your very own thoughts.
while formative and compelling,
they are not in the seat of power—you are.
they do not characterise you, but if left unattended
they can influence your feelings and actions
unnoticed.

thoughts are just thoughts and your marvelous
brain can examine them, try them on for size
and if they don't fit just right they can be
replaced by newer and more intentional ones.

(this process becomes more difficult, however
the longer these thoughts run free.)

today, if your thoughts are telling you lies
such as worthless, wasted, or weak
rather than running,
grab those thoughts with both hands
hold them up to the light to discover their flaws.

toss out the bad
enhance the good,
—and just forget some of them altogether.

but whatever, remember
that you are in the driver's seat.
you are in command.

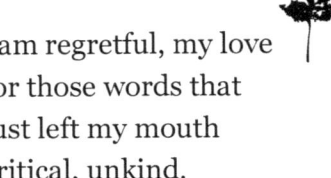

i am regretful, my love
for those words that
just left my mouth
critical, unkind.

something that i had not
yet noticed bounced
off my own heart, unexpected
and targeted yours instead
—for this i must earnestly apologise.

i will stop now, take space and listen
grapple with this clue i have been given
find the culprit in *my* heart

instead of continuing to ask
you to bear the brunt of an
issue that is mine.

> — projecting our issues onto others
> is a destroyer of relationships.

we wander through grass to table cement
and sit on the same side
watching seagulls whirl on wind
above green-green hills and sparkling sea

and you talk—and i listen
soaking in your thoughts
and later we philosophise

until you walk around to other side
and lay long-tall frame down on bench
with sighs

and peering above table between
all i can see is nose and eyes-shut face
and you talk—and i listen
and i smell the grass and feel the breeze

and at this time there is no place else
on God's green earth i would choose to be
breathing soft in this moment fully present
moving little lest you, young colt
should startle and bolt, spirited

and you talk—and i listen
the treasure of mothering a grown-up son
and you talk—and i listen thankful
and my heart fills brim-full to running over
with peace

you are caught in a tangle
a maze of worry and unease
sending you scattered down the path
forgetting which direction to go
whether you last turned right or left
bewildered.

you stop
        and turn
                and realise
that the walls that surround are not
as solid as they seem.

as you examine them
you begin to see patterns—
swirls and angles assembled

and realise then that a hedge full
of bushes and vines does not
a prison make.
that freedom is entirely possible
and is even close at hand.

and as you compare the logic available
in this moment to the chaos of the last
you realise that slowing right down
and facing your fears
has shown they were not
as dangerous as you supposed.

that the threats, perceived
shadows out of the corner of your eye,
were not impenetrable
as you assumed before you turned
to face them head-on.

then you sit right down
place hands on hedge
unravel some branches here
detangle some vines over there
and you slip right through the
space

and find that you in fact
are now no longer bound.

she sat in the front turning
her head of gray
back and forth, back and forth
waiting for a break in traffic.

in the passenger's seat sat a
faithful friend as invested
in the process as she.

back and forth, back and forth
in perfect unison—together.

and i imagine that the passenger's
tail wagged a bit when a break
in cars they finally found.

sometimes
the most powerful thing a person can do
is simply to refuse.

refuse to go down without a fight.
refuse the fear that lurks within
that sense of guilt or shame.

refuse to listen to that cycle
that plays now on repeat:
not good enough.
too much.
useless.
unworthy.

to pick themselves up
to hold on to the last shred of light.
strength is discovered in places such as these
resiliency formed.

it is not the denial of pain or its cause
but the recognition
the acceptance
that what is—just is

and then choosing
nay, *refusing*
to become defined by the pain.

they never tell you when you hold
your own soft babe
that the pain that might pierce their heart
can shatter yours as well

that love and sorrow are so intermingled, woven
that you often cannot feel the one without the other
always cradled close you carry them in a satchel
next to your very soul

wind lashes, sand stings
the spray of the sea arrives unexpected
and booms against the rocks.

i lean into the power of the howling blast.

watching the crashing waves,
they speak to my heart
of things that are greater than i

and of One whom i can trust
to keep those i love secure
—even amidst the tempest.

she told me to accept what i was feeling
all that i felt without judgment, and this
i tried to do. until i realised there was
one item i was long conditioned to ignore
or control, but never-ever allow to run free.

i thought that anger was just a downward
spiral into hate and rage. i thought it inhibited
forgiveness and peace, and 'not ladylike'
was deeply ingrained as well.

but my head has learned that anger has
its place, its own type of service
and bears a scent that must be exhaled
as part of a story of injustice identified.

and she is welcome here
for others—and even for ourselves
yes, this is acceptable too.

so, i breathed in deep and shut my eyes
and listened in the dark to what anger
had to say.

and she began to communicate

louder and more convincingly than any voice
i had ever heard: "this was not right.
this should not have happened."

and i found i most heartily agreed.

and the fire blazed and burned and for maybe
the first time, i embraced the heat and watched
what happened next . . .

instead of consuming me she began to devour
things like misplaced guilt and should-have-dones
and sadness with her searing blue-white flame.

and her sister, grief, nodded, stood
and clapped her hands at last.

certain anger is not meant to be tamed
but to burn white hot until at last released.
so let it roar and turn to ash that which
sparked the heat within your chest
consuming pain and shame and horror
of what was and is until there is peace
and embers flicker and finally grow cold
—satiated.

and you will look and say "that pain, it
squeezed my soul for far too long and
sucked oxygen from gasping lungs"

but now that anger is free to do
the purifying task it was designed
to accomplish all along
you are finally free.

—anger has its proper place and function.

love first blooms fresh and sparkling with dew
fragile like a tiny shoot that must be
tended and nourished with care.

but over time, oh the places that love can grow!

roots deep in the soul, souls intertwined
bonded together by memories, experiences
and adventures shared, home.

when you can say "remember when" and talk for hours
or sit in content not speaking at all.

when you can catch one glance and comprehend
the depth and breadth of meaning therein.

when you have chosen daily for years
this person, this relationship, this life
then you will know more of what love is
what it can be—and what it is not.

love is holy work and work it is
but a treasure beyond price it becomes
        when protected
                nourished
                        cherished
when consistently chosen over time
worth every moment invested
as gold.

the worst thing about fear
is that it steals your todays
with thoughts of something
that may never-ever happen

leading to a life of moments lost
imprisoned by a ghastly
thief of time and tranquility
who continually whispers lies.

—beware of its ways.

if you, my friend, carry a cup of tea
across a crowded room
and on the way your arm is bumped
by a thoughtless person or two

then out of the cup will slosh
not water or juice or coffee
—but tea

your cup may be paper
or styrofoam
or ceramic
or glass
or the finest porcelain even

it might be decorated bright
or be the plainest of plain
—the outside of the cup
is not what matters

because if tea is what's inside
then when knocked
(as teacups often are)
then tea is what will slosh

and i ask you this (as i ask my own self too)
what is it that splashes out
when you become jarred
or bumped or pushed
a little too hard

what is in *your* cup
that might spill out
all over whoever
happens to be near?

being jostled from time
to time
is unavoidable
but you can be in charge
of what is inside

> — this is an important matter to monitor and
> ascertain *(metaphor from society at large).*

a flame flickers in the darkness
bouncing shadows off the wall
darkness shrinks back, startled.

it only takes one small flame to do this
because light is stronger
and darkness will always recede
when light is in the room.

remember this when hope is dim
and joy has fled.

the dark, while dense and imposing
muscles flexing and intentions clear,
cannot withstand even
the very least of flames—and magnifies
the presence of light simply by existing.

so allow the dark to enhance the light
and focus on the flame.

protect it, feed it
and the darkness *will* flee
every-single-time.

      — let there be light.

wouldn't it be amazing
if we could raise our children
with perfection

but instead, just like a thousand
generations have before
we must muddle along

offering them the best of what we can
and living an example of how to
do things a little bit better
each and every day.

for perhaps a year or even three
i wondered—not fully in doubt, because i had
too much evidence gathered through
a lifetime of experience

that you are real
that you are good
that a life spent with you
is a life worth living

but all the discourses of all the thinking
and reasoning and logic of others
did make some part of me wonder
even if just a bit—and it kept me from you

from being able to fully appreciate you
to talk openly with you
and while my mind did not admit it,
my heart struggled to fully trust.

but then—at the right and honest time
after i had grown in ways i now appreciate
even if i do not fully understand
and while nothing else has really changed

—the veil in my dimly lit heart was raised
and now i see you clear again
now i feel you near

and now—even on difficult days,
i am once again confident in the depths

of my heart and soul

and while i know the road
will have patches of uneven ahead
this one thing i understand
better than ever before

and i say like that woman in the desert
so very long ago:

that you are the One-who-sees, really sees, me
you understand the core
of a very human heart
a heart like mine

there is nothing that escapes your gaze
and you have all these situations
securely, firmly, safely held
in your loving hand.

i do not care what you have heard
from the lips of society cold
you are not your pain
your shame or your despair.
no, these are just things—they don't define

they are simply a cloak you wear from time to time
when the temperature drops
or even by habit when sun still shines

but as seasons and styles change
so will the cloak that you wear
and you—yes, you, my friend
can make this cloak your helper

take it in your hands, reconfigure the cut and fit
fashion it instead into something beautiful
and worthwhile

then take charge of when you wear it
for these things that happened *to* you
were never back then
       and are never right now
           and never will they ever be
who you *are*.

      — do not wear pain and trauma as an identity.

there are things in this world that horrify
that can invade our space in a single breath

but there is also a tree with yellow leaves
piercing through the gray of the day

i bring you my list of worries
and fears, transactional even,
unrefined. i know you
will listen because i am like
a child and you my parent
and infinitely more besides.

but in the process of telling
you come close, and while i don't
see your form or examine your
face, i know the feel of you well
how you comfort and hold my heart
and soothe my mind with light.

and i stop and realise that while
i still don't know the future
or how i will handle today
and while i long to see things
miraculous and dazzling
(and at times i have) that your nearness
is really all i need for now.

knowing that you are close
and care more than anyone ever
has or ever possibly could
invites me into things like peace
and joy and calms the waves within.

so i take your hand, always outstretched
and hang on tight again.

i will take the next step different
more sure since you are my help

and even if my hand grows weary
of holding on—you will never let go of mine.

if you want to heal
you must feel the feelings.
while millions of humans before us
have tried to escape this
—there is just no other way.

they will bubble and brew
and expand until they escape
some way or the other, regardless

so, while highly uncomfortable,
let them out slowly
like the hiss of a bottle of fizz.

it is better than bottling them up
for years
uncomfortably tight

only to explode with force
or debilitate
despite all your best efforts
to minimise.

this is the difficult work
that is healing.
this takes courage

but this is the way to freedom
from those things
you would rather avoid

that hold you captive
while you exhaustively pretend
to be okay

but imagine what it could be like
to finally
be free.

> — paying attention to what you feel is an
> incredibly vital step towards healing.

you do not
look like me
sound like me
talk like me
think like me
act like or
dream like me.
still, we are the same.

both made in the image
of One greater than
our imaginations could
generate, our differences
inconsequential because
we both come from and
in our deepest of longings
migrate back towards
the very same things.

and i am the less if i do not
see you the same way that
i see me—perfectly
made but imperfectly
patterned—just like myself.
pricelessly
wonderfully
chaotically
joyously
human.

someone i admire was asked
how they came through the hardest
times and made it to the other side.

the answer was simple, they paid
attention to beauty and no matter
what else came their way

beauty was always there, always
available, always free—if someone
takes the pause to see
that while famine, war and shame exist
there is also *this*.

no matter what the world throws our way
no matter what happens within
the confines of our frame

there might be a tree of brilliant yellow
right outside the window or a cat curled
tight upon our lap for warmth, or a bird
serenading in the garden just because it can
with dew upon the daisies in tall grass.

so, while there is evil and ugly
[and make no mistake, there is]
there is still always, now and forever
always also *this*.

the earth holds its breath, waiting
for calm, for hope, for belly laughter
for rest.

today may appear dark, but
while the earth keeps spinning and
the sun sits in the sky, dawn will
always, always come, constant.
scientists, politicians, philosophers
spiritual leaders and poets can all agree on this.

i don't know about you
but my brain tries to resist
sadness and doesn't want
to listen
to its quiet, insistent roar.

perhaps the mind is convinced
that if it pretends that sadness
doesn't exist—
it will 'poof' it away.

let me tell you now, however,
that little fox of a thought
will consume the whole henhouse
if allowed to run free.

grief is not something that
will dissipate unattended.
it is a wound that requires
tending and gentle care
for healing to softly come
and will fester increasingly
without acknowledgement.

> — letting sadness breathe is
> uncomfortable, but necessary.

i remember feeling fragile during summer
perhaps more so with the scarlet in the trees.
so, when winter came, i closed the window
waiting for the surge of cold to pass

and cozy in my blanket, cup of
tea in hand—i pause.

not peacefully at first, because accepting
the need for rest is perhaps the most
difficult but important part of healing.

even the trees know that seasons change
and healing comes
the sun will shine
and all things bloom again.

— the need for rest is not failure or weakness.

i leave the pegs on the clothesline, waiting
instead of gathering them in
like some would maintain
that i should do.

and today they playfully cavort
twisting in the wind, merrily colored.
hanging on for dear life—and succeeding
just as they were designed
on this otherwise dismal day.

and i imagine if i were a peg
that this is what i would prefer.

i could be lying safely inside
but in a box, restrained

but i would rather embrace the gale
and *dance*.

> — it is far better to experience life
> than to be cloistered for longevity.

if you cannot move
feet planted solid and fast
stuck in the mud and muck
you can at least still lean

lean into the direction that you next want to go
the place where fields of grace await
do not lean back in remembrance of the place
that you have been.

it is fine to gather bouquets of lessons learned
but do not go back to the site of your scars
do not seek the presence
of the things that did this

that was *then*
this is *now.*
so in this moment, lean

lean strong and intentional towards grace
grace for others too, but mostly towards
the grace you never offered *you*

a child throws tantrums because they do not
know how to identify a need
it's not really about a fizzy or a biscuit
or not putting on their shoes

it's about the need for rest or comfort
or the calming of a mind overstimulated

you have grace for this—but you struggle
with grace for you

i do not say this to add to any guilt or shame
but to gently point to that doorway, that portal
that leads the way towards grace

softly beckoning
gently drawing
you can follow her there if you choose.

childish faces from time past
cherished grins and beloved frames
—how is it that a single photo
can take your breath away?

take you right back to the details
of that moment and to a place
where you miss these people
who still exist, but who have

grown and changed and if possible
have made you love them even more.
yet it would be inexplicably lovely
to go back, to spend even one hour with

who they also used to be. to pull them
onto your lap and cuddle once again.
to listen to their chatter on the events
of the day, of what went right and

what went wrong. to be the one who gets
to hear these precious things. to smell
their skin and capture that moment in
greater detail once again because you

blinked and now they're grown and
while you wouldn't change the person
they've become, you also miss the one
they used to be.

you are allowed to
walk away from
that argument
that conversation that disturbs
that relationship that damages
that situation that steals your sleep.

you can change
your definition of victory or success
from gaining the upper hand
to protecting and maintaining
your very own peace.

you do not need to ruminate
just let it go. let it slide right off
like a non-stick surface and take
back what is one of the very few things
that truly is your own—your thoughts.

you decide what is important
what takes up residence between your ears.
no one else can do that *to* you
—you get to choose.

and you may be surprised at what
arguments, conversations, relationships
or situations you can handle
—once you have chosen
to foster peace.

when i was young, i wanted to
study the stars—until i discovered
that math would be required

but the wonder of staring into starry skies
has never waned, it is still just
as magical as when i was nine.

that pulling of the soul into
mystery, the unfathomable
enormity of it all.

something that cannot be held
within two hands, like the wind,
like the waves—

but even greater still. we think
we are wise, but our minuscule
brains cannot contain

the vastness of space billowing out
beyond our ability to explain,
inspiring stories eloquent

of adventures in unknown. but when
i stare into the starry night i cannot
speak—and think about the face of God.

you can choose to let
the judgement of others go.
let it roll out of your head
and drip down your limbs
until it falls to the ground,
soaks into the soil
—and vanishes.

she walked
towards me
arms so full
that her face
was unseen

and in her grasp
both fresh
and fragrant
were not the
cares of this world

or pain experienced
(i know her well,
she had access
to these)

but instead
in her arms
bursting and
barely contained

were blooms
of softness
and grace
and a riot
of colour
such as i have
never before seen
because

on her journey
she had not
held on
to troubles
or pain

no, she
had hunted
wildflowers.

out beyond where your thoughts may wander
is a field of grass so green that all you want to do
is lay down on soft blades silent.

there are many days you never reach this space
this place of quiet and rest because for you at least,
rest involves discipline:

quieting the mind
listening with whole heart and being,
cutting through layers of distraction
all the prisms of a rainbow bright.

dialling down
heart-slowing focus
is not your natural state,
but oh, the peace you find
when you make the effort
take the time
avoid all possible detours
to arrive at this healing space.

this is the place where problems lose their power
and what only an hour or so ago felt insurmountable
is now seen through the perspective of peace.

this is where you feel closest to God
where you get to walk with him in the cool of the day
picking flowers here
wading through peaceful streams there

and laying down once again
on the softest green-green grass
to rest

      — seek this space devotedly and often.

i know it has been a while
and you are tired of seeing that person
you love struggle. they are tired, too.

but please remember that while
"just get on with it" works for some,
a person who has experienced trauma
still wears it within their frame.

it is not an experience to be forgotten,
it is an internal fracture
as a result of the experience.

you would not tell someone whose leg
was broken to just get back to walking.
the injury of your person is unseen
and they have likely tried to 'walk'
on it far too long already.

healing takes time—and support,
physio for the heart and understanding
as a dressing for the soul.
there will come a time for them
to move forward, but it will likely not be when
you think they should

and they might always have a limp.
but they will grow and will be stronger
in other remarkable ways
—with time.

when i was younger
i worried about who may
or may not invite me to
the table. i feared rejection
and saw loneliness waiting
in the wings.

(and to be completely honest
the older me does still somewhat
worry about this as well.)

but my head now knows
that difference is an exciting
thing. we are all not 'same'
for a reason.

diversity inspires great legends
the painter's brush
the minstrel's song
the adventurer's map.

beauty is a thrilling and
varied thing and there really
is enough to go around.

so if i am not your cup of tea
please drink coffee instead.
this is fine and between us we
make a much more interesting
and vibrant occasion for us all.

as i sat in the room with my most loved ones
and played the game of *remember when,* i realised
that the most treasured things in life
aren't the perfect, either in the living—or the retelling

but the memories, the most precious parts
of the story of us are the things
that didn't go as planned.

like how the youngest was sick when we travelled through bangkok
—every. single. time.

and how we walked with tired limbs for hours
to find transport after the new year's firework display
off dubai's *burj khalifa* that only lasted five minutes.

and that we almost lost each other in another new year's eve
crush, clinging desperately to each other's hands on park street,
calcutta. somewhat horrific, but laughing in the end.

and then there's the crazy old man who screamed at us to get back
from the edge of the grand canyon even though there was no way we
could have fallen.

or the too-hot-to-sleep nights in fiji
when all the neighbours would sing
harmonies floating in balmy air.

and when dad thought that there was a gas station ahead but there
wasn't, yet we made it on fumes to the ancient glacier on the west
coast of the south island of new zealand.

so many stories of adventure survived around the world—together
incredible shared beauty that marks and feeds our corporate soul.

it is not the amusement parks or fleeting pleasures
but the stories of adversity leisurely spoken of in our reminiscing.
these are the things that bind us, our familial togetherness.

priceless narratives reminding us
we have really lived—and often thrived.

the cracks in our lives that are 'just ours', they make us strong.
shared adversity seals our hearts in priceless ways
in a bond that no one else can quite appreciate.

so, the next time things don't go quite as planned
instead of stress, embrace.
gather the 'not quite' fiercely
hold it close to your chest

let it grow rich in memory, and smile
because it's all the golden cracks that hold us together
that embody the most beautiful whole.

i have watched you for years
watched over you from the
moment of your first breath.
delighted at your first word
first step.

i have done my best
to guard you
keep you safe,
while also aspiring
to instil a sense of
wonder at the world around
and an understanding
of your importance in it.

your talents, abilities,
a joy to you,
a gift of fresh air to others.

but now it is up to you,
i cannot walk your path
cannot dream your dreams
hold your hand, plan your way.

this is part of letting go
and you must take the reins.
—and i
must not block the way.

joy is not elsewhere, far off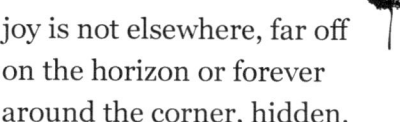
on the horizon or forever
around the corner, hidden.

this frantic quest may take you
far and wide, probing distant
galaxies

but when you find her
i think you will be astonished
that she was nearby all along.
here.

    right now.

        in this place.

you had this idea that you could go out
into the large wide world and somehow
be able to bear all that you came across:
the joys, the pains, the labour futile

but the moments that made it all worth it,
were fewer and further between
than you ever imagined

and you gave and you poured out
ladles of water here and there
into the endless everywhere

still you were surprised that you became dry
shrivelled as walnuts do
and you had nothing left with which to wash
your own cracked skin
or cleanse from your heart the ongoing struggle
of other people's pain

you knew that 'heartless' was never a name
you could sew into your skin,
yet your heart desensitised bit by bit, shattered

carrying other people's pain
is a habit unsustainable.
this is not calloused, you see—but vital

for if this habit continues it will only harm *you*
and will do nothing to alleviate their suffering

so you retreated for a time to ponder
to lick your wounds, to heal
and discovered that even though 'empathy'
is your unspoken name

this must be extended to yourself *first*.
then you can offer its balm around,
this pain is theirs, not yours, to bear.

so now as you sit with others
whose hearts have broken
you allow the feelings to ebb and flow like tide
and you remember, while pain is a thing
that must be felt—you can release it as well

— it is not possible to carry other people's pain

the fog rolls in soft and comforting.
tendrils of mist whisper: "this is okay.
you are safe, protected. you do not need
to venture out of my embrace.

the time will come, but not just yet.
so curl up on cushion soft and wait
for me to leave

and take the gift i offer now—of rest."

there you stand, dipping in your
toe to test the temperature.

is it too hot, or too cold
too challenging, or too tame
too tiring, or worth the effort
—or are you just afraid?

meanwhile life is passing
you by, so just jump right in
—the water is fine.

i have spent too much time
in the land of in-between
not really happy, but not
really sad. making it through
the day, but not taking the
time to fan into flame the
spark of joy that lives
within, tired.

while the influence is less
than in times past,
this is the habit i strive to
unlearn completely before
any more life passes me by.

and to do that, i must remember
to feel. not just flatten and ignore
those emotions that dwell within
but allow them to breathe
and speak
and listen.

for while the mind might fear the
message they bring, no breadth
of emotion has ever killed me yet.

no, the real hazard is that land
of in-between that soullessly
steals away days one-by-one
depressed.

and whatever life has thrown my way
—and it has given its best—
i still get to choose where
to reside.

in-between is a place
i will always determine to leave
for it is a thief.
its travel brochure is titled 'safe'
—but it lies.

i had to gather myself together
to leave my home that day.
tired, teeming paths and stifling heat
my soul thirsty for softer things.

relieved to locate a seat on the train,
both my daughter and i. my weary gaze
finally left the floor, wandering up
to a woman sitting across.

she was so very soft and serene, at peace,
unremarkably dressed
nothing particularly of note
and yet—in absolute stillness and assurance
she held my gaze.

her face radiated things like:
take heart, it is going to be okay, you are
never alone—and, be patient,
this too shall pass.

these thoughts permeated my mind
and i sighed in deep and knew
this moment was profound and
gifted for my good

our stop was announced. we rose in silence
within that city's fierce hum
and i filed the encounter away
—private, sacred, mine.

when years later i finally spoke of these things
one lazy afternoon, my daughter nodded matter-of-fact
"oh, i remember her, too"

and she used the word i had been hesitant to say.
that while some must announce "do not be afraid"
other angels come quiet and unexpected
on places like calcutta trains

proclaiming hope-filled things
and peace on earth today.

there is a space that is miraculous
where the things that were dead
gasp and come alive once again.
and once you have seen this
experienced this
—you will never breathe the same.

sit with me beside the sea
and let us watch the waves
and maybe you'll remember
there is power beyond
your own frame of reference
and fantastic beauty
to be found
all around

and this disengagement
you have worn as
part of survival long
may start to fade
if we sit here and
watch together
in hope
and wait.

when fragile
comes to call
a visit has often
recently occurred
by cousin *'should'*
who whispers,
foul breath upon
our necks, that
mistakes *should* not be made, or
the responsibility
of the happiness of others
should be ours to bear,
or we *should* not have needs
of our own.

he is an ungrateful
guest and the only
'should' we need
take notice of then
is that we *should*
show him the door.
then shut it firm
and tight, breathe
deep of air without
his stench and make
choices without
his crafty, filthy lies.

i would have never wished
for you to go through
the waters that you did.

i wish i could have been
stronger than the wind,
more forceful than the
waves. that i could have
calmed the storm with
a single powerful word.

but you have made it
to the shore, you have
crawled up on the sand,
and while you may need
to rest there for some time,
that is fine.

for while you are tired now
the onslaught has shaped you
in spectacular ways
and you have had edges smoothed
a new shape formed
that would have taken years,
if ever, without the storm.

we always know when hunting season arrives
as flocks of ducks and geese migrate to sanctuary
flying low like arrows
over our roof
squawking loud

i have heard this is not to announce their arrival
but to spur on the one who is in front
expending the most energy in formation:

"keep going
you've got this
we're here with you"
they proclaim

until the one in front tires
then they take turns
and cheer the next one on as well
as they make their way towards places safe
together

  — lessons from nature

carrying stones so heavy you have
stumbled too long, too far to maintain balance.
you have done your best to heal

and while the finish line may still seem
so long, so far away, you have come an incredible
distance—i want to remind you of this.

what is it that holds you back
from all the things that you
ever wanted?

is it the concept of change,
that dive into the unknown,
the potential risk of fall?

i know that you have all
you need, have prepared
for this for long

and whether or not the motions
are smooth or need correction
on the way

do not ponder the fear, my love,
just focus on the dive.

the storm is rising, forecasting
days of torrential rain ahead.

i walk down by the beach and
lean into the wind, struggling
to stay upright, grinning at other
humans as we pass each other brave

hair flying, clothing dancing.

then i glimpse the perfect
sight of hope in the face of
impending tempest.

sails rippling and smiles wide,
they run towards water and choose
the elements as their friend.

laughing at its efforts, they
harness instead. letting wind carry
them across ocean in pure,
intentional joy.

i stop, sit, and watch a while,
ponytail whips my face,
and i welcome the challenge stirring within

that this is how to face the season ahead.
not retreating, not hiding, not afraid,
but shoulders squared, becoming
the beauty within the storm.

you do not complete me
in fact, no one else is meant to.

this idea of completion
is a killer of relationships,
unrealistic in expectation
and execution.

it's entirely unreasonable
to expect *you* to fill the void
that makes *me* whole.

my insecurities, my issues,
my healing required. these are
mine to bear, not yours,
not corporately ours.

but complement each other we do.
we fit together hand and glove
because we have executed adjustments
repeatedly—large and small

done the mahi[1], put in the effort
and have chosen each other again
every. single. day.

we are two imperfect people
pursuing wholeness—together
and loving each other

---

1   Māori word that speaks to the hard work necessary to get the job done

wholeheartedly
along the way.

and because of this, my cup is full.
and when you are near
or even far away
i feel the completeness
we have each found
and share
together.

the daylight slips away
and songbirds sweetly sing
the day to close

and you, who used to
fear the dark, breathe deep
and relish in the hush

joining nature in her rhythms
tranquil, for all must
slumber and refresh

and tomorrow's troubles
are not today's and need
to keep their place.

and night is nothing to be
feared when a heart chooses
peaceful and content.

do not gaze long on the bottom of the jar
that reveals scarcity, lack.

empty is not there to appropriate your
thoughts and transform into fear.

it simply means there is room to be filled
so imagine . . .
what could that substance be?

      —you get to choose.

as i contemplate the grief
the loss
the crushing down
the tumble
the resistance
the death of who i was
into the resurrection of who i am

i remember back to the beginning
when i would have given anything
to simply jump the chasm of grief
to the other side

and say "ah ha" to loss
"i have foiled you
i laugh at your intention
you have not got me yet."

this would have thrilled me then,
but now i look back and gaze
down at my own two hands,
the things that these hands and heart
can hold and the things that they
have made

because you would not have
convinced me in the middle
that this could at all be true
—but now i treasure the things
pain has gifted me

things like:
"you will keep breathing,
you will stand up once again,
this journey will have an end"

and what it was like in the midst
of darkness thick to see
the very first crack
the tear in the black
when light came through again

the morning sun breaks
through the clouds
after days
and days
of rain

and you recall
the beauty
once again
that is possible

and all of
those things
that troubled
and stole
your sleep

seem to vanish
like mist
in life-giving
rays of scarlet

i want you to know today tomorrow
and every day in-between
that i am solid.

i am the rock beneath your feet
the steady for your hands,
i am the washer away of hurt
from you and from those you love too.

i want you to know that i will never ever ask you
to suck your soul dry
i will never value others above you.
i am big enough to gather round and nestle close
every human heart—and yours is not less
valuable than any one of these.

i am enough for you,
i am deeper and wilder and more expansive
than you could ever dream.

i will not let you down
blinking out of existence at inconvenient times,
i want you to know that i will endure
i am here

i am permanent
when all else fades i will not,
i will not fail you

— letter from God

i feel the breeze stir
slight and soft against my skin
and reflect that the winds of
change also move slow
in this circumstance that aches

as breath catches in my chest
and i long with all that i am
to move heavens and earth
for this.

but mid-sigh, i lift my eyes
to treetops waving.
lacy fingers stirred by a force
in the heavens that i cannot feel
with feet firmly planted
on the ground.

and oh, how the branches dance!

and my heart remembers
there is more than
my limited experience,
my point of view,
perception

that change has a force of its own
and God does things that my finite outlook
often cannot see

and the beat in my chest
joins in, slowly at first

but as i stay in that moment hush
my heart begins
to slip off her shoes
and lifts up her feet
to dance.

there is warmth
hot drink and fire
just inside the door.
you see it through the window
standing outside in falling snow, sodden

what is it that hesitates
that keeps hands down at sides
feet unmoving
shallow breathing?

you want all that is bright
and meaningful and cordial
on the other side
—i see the longing there

what will it take to lift the latch
to come in out of cold
heart frozen but able to be softened
mended?

but still you stand
and i realise . . . that in itself
is courage

—you're simply getting ready

come to the place that is rest softly. you need not
shout it loud. it is fine if you can only stumble in
through the door, but just make sure you
come.

as you take off your shoes and lay by streams
of peaceful waters, you will find that all of the
striving has made you weary, more than you
realised, and that quiet is productive, too.

and it is good to linger in this space where you
can let those burdens go, where you can evaluate
what is yours to bear—or not
and which flowers you will gather,
what memories you wish to make

and the priorities you will intentionally choose
once you arise again.

and as your mind calms to the peaceful rhythm of
the brook, simply let thoughts go and you will
find rest for your soul

—and just *be*.

when you put a seed
down into soil deep
you must wait—
because it will
never germinate, grow
if you keep digging it
up to check on its
progress.

i know this is hard
but it's just the way
that it is with all
things plant—and
most everyone's
heart as well.

you must simply
gently water,
make sure
there is light
—and wait.

just because you are
below the surface
surrounded by
water entire

does not mean you have sunk
to the bottom, irretrievably
entangled in rocky cave.

you might just be
mere metres beneath
the cover of waves

and only a few small
strokes of fluttering feet
from the pure air that sustains

so do not peer down
into the depths, discouraged.
instead look up to the light
seek the warmth of the sun

be encouraged by its nearness
and you will break free from
the smother of a space
you were only intended to visit

and return to the habitat
you were born into. a place
where you can freely live
and breathe and flourish.

in the spirit of transparency
i want to let you know
that while i may appear
sometimes at least
put together without
i am always learning
to be put together
within.

no matter what your
impression of me may be
i still have things to learn
i still have spots blind

i still work towards
kindness and ever-always
towards general put-togetherness.

i may look sorted outside
but some days i am
rumble-tumbling on the in

fighting insecurities
battling emotions
sorting out my
frequently tangled
thoughts.

i keep thinking that someday
maybe i will arrive

but perhaps it is better this way.
it keeps me humble

invites me to have short
accounts with myself and
others and consistently teaches
a multitude of helpful things.

so if this is in any way
like you are too, i see you.

let us nod and offer quiet, kind
looks of understanding as we meet
upon the street—and i am open
to high-fives, too.

you hang your head in
sorrow because you do
not know the crown
unseen that sits upon it.

you do not remember
there is a life lived
full and wild and free,
and experiences to draw upon

and that your worth has nothing
to do with what you *do*,
but with who you were

when you knelt
alone on bathroom floor
before your hardest day

when your hope
was dim, uncertainty
all around

and who you have become
as you kept on walking
anyway, trying to be faithful
even though broken.

you, yes you, are still here
and you are worthy of things
that are good

of life still to be lived
of gifts unexpected yet to be given.

so, do not give up, my dear
raise your head, straighten
crooked crown, know when
to accept assistance along the
way and remember
—you are glorious.

the walls loom high
insurmountable.
and while i know
you make a way
i am not sure that you will.

you part the sea
you flatten walls
you move mountains
—and you have
for me. but in this instance

the battle has gone on
far too long and i am
tired. and while i know that you
do everything in your time
i wish your time were now.

but then it occurs to me
that focusing on the problem
is always exhausting
plotting the solution

is overwhelming
and that life is best lived
today, now. so i stop

and breathe, extend my hands
and remember that in this moment
in time you are right here, always

and that no matter how long
or high or wide this wall
—right now, even now
with you i am on holy ground.

how did she know
after twelve long years
of suffering
that this

this one man
with nothing special
about his features, his frame
was worth struggling towards
through the crowd
in order to touch his hem?

how, after all that time
of adversity, discomfort, alone
did she have faith enough to believe
that something extraordinarily small
yet so difficult to implement
was worth the persistence it took
to lean into hope once again?

and she pushed through the crowd
and touched the hem.

are you getting to know
the you that is emerging
wings furled and wet
from cocoon that transforms?

you are different,
not the same as the one
who entered change's
hallowed halls

what did you learn within?
did you discover meaning there,
how not to feel lost?

did the cocoon communicate soft
the truth that you do not need
to rush to metamorphosis
to repair?

these things take all the time they need,
patient.

you have wings developed
and opening them takes practice
but remember, once you soar above
you will find your way

to be accepted
to be included
to be known for who we are
this, the deepest longing of
every human heart

yet we spend most
of our time distracted, busy
getting on to the next thing
the next task
the next entertainment
the next thing we *should* do

ignoring the inner call
towards connection
and we wilt
    and we wither away
        alone in the crowd.

throw off the bonds
that society has fabricated
of how we must conform, fit in

go for a walk in a meadow
sit under a tree
look up at the leaves
notice the light that filters there
the quiet humming of the air
the gentle way it nuzzles skin
and contemplate for a while.

there, within creation
you will find connection
in the rhythms of nature
and remember that *you*
are also linked to Holy.

this, a balm for your heart
a freeing of your mind
and a clarion reminder
that you are already
known
and loved.

once you can breathe free again
reenter humanity and remember . . .

connection is best found
within simplicity
and by being authentic
with who you truly are.

       —you cannot find real connection without this.

i will not lie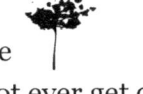
you may not ever get over this
but you can get through it

one foot in front of other
one decision at a time.

and i will not sugar-coat it
the going may be more arduous
than you ever imagined

but if you keep on moving
you will find that walking becomes
easier with each passing mile and
the gravity that pulls you back is less

and less, until one day you will realise
just how far you have roamed

and that experience monstrous
is but a dot in distance.

your wounds, while scarred, have
healed now and very seldom ache

and your heart that felt like boulder
heavy is buoyant, drawing in the sun.

and you will lift your head and gasp
with the freshness of the air in lungs
that struggled once to breathe

and your eyes, blinded previously
by waterfalls of tears, will drink in
beauty once again.

i will not minimise the things that you
are feeling now . . .

but i can assure you without a shadow
of a doubt, that as you keep on going
and moving
and breathing
and living
you can
      and will
           get through.

it is no small thing
to wake with sunshine
in your heart

to feel fresh morning rays
and anticipate the day to come,
to experience peace in the early
misty light

this is my ardent wish for you:
that the nightmares are gone and
cannot bleed into the day.
that the things that are past
are historical alone,
and do not pertain to your present.

you have worked so very hard and
come incredibly far, and while this
thought might sound insignificant
to some

to you it would indicate healing,
deep and wide and strong
and free.

so may this morning arrive soon
and may you face that day
and the next
and the next
from a place of rest.

i believe in possibility
and i trust this day
will come,
even if *you* cannot
—yet.

i do not need to defend you
giver-of-life, bringer-of-peace,
you can stand on your own two feet
and have been doing this far longer

than i have been in existence.
but i do implore you, beseech
you, to show yourself both kind
and strong to this person i love

who needs your light and life
and right now thinks that you
are but a dopamine rush in
my brain and do not really
exist.

you have chosen to make yourself
un-seeable, unexplainable
and this generation who have witnessed
hypocrisy indeed in the frame of your name
have chosen science and things proven
as their source of wisdom and truth.

and while i cannot blame them really,
i also cannot deny the presence of
things that can't be seen
since you have made known to me
impossible peace and joy in the midst
of the worst life has to offer

you have walked beside me as i
drank from streams
of life and love and joy

you have been my light in dark places,
and put strength within my bones.
my companion constant,
who has never let me go.

as you have done for me and still
every day do, please shine your light
in a way that cannot be explained
or missed

and let this heart tattered
understand that you will do this
for them too.

you ask why you need
to forgive when you are not
the one who committed
the deed, that caused the pain
that left an indelible mark.

and i smile and reply soft,
that forgiveness is not about
them, it is critically more
about *you*.

it does not excuse what they
did, but rather protects your
already hurting heart from
further disrepair, from
bitterness growing deep
down into bones.

forgiveness means that
freedom for you
is on the way
and heralds
its approach loud.

there it is just beneath the surface.
be patient as it blows
away dust, brushes out
cobwebs sticky, and
your heart will
sparkle again.

the mountain soars above
drawing close her cloak
of cloud white. you wonder
what she thinks of you from
her far off, towering heights.

"i am still here" she whispers
in your ear. "i am proof that solid
things remain."

on our last holiday we panned for gold:
tipped water in, shook, gently poured
released dirt, sand, and pebbles
over and over until
all that was left
were small flecks

that sit now in a
vial on a shelf, a reminder
of a time well spent
—together.

how much like us this is . . .

every time we dip into the waters
more and more of the things we
brought with us from before
filter away.

every time we feel the shake of circumstances,
the grit surrounding us loosens and floats,
cast aside.

every time we address troubles and choose
each other once again each and every day,
the sand separates
and departs.

and in this patient, steady process
we have found much more
than specks of gold.

we have found nuggets solid
and veins precious running through
and throughout

the treasure
that makes up us and
grows more evident each
day that we pan this life
—together.

other people's expectations
of how you should walk
talk, dress, relate, perform
and many other things
are not your burden to bear.

do not allow them to cage
you in. for while some of
their advice might be of use
you get to choose entire
what that is or what it is not.

to accept their unfettered
opinions without discernment
creates nothing more than
a prison that keeps you
bound up tight

while you are the one who holds
the lock and the key. so do not
look for approval from those
who would rather see you
bound.

in those meaningless interactions
with those who pass you by, you
also can decide how to interpret
their glances—as either
judgement or approval.

and why do you often not even
consider the source, looking for
admiration from those you do
not even value? keep a tight rein
on whose opinions matter

place yourself high upon that list.
evaluate the expectations of others
and if you choose to, stretch out
capable hands—and let
                them
        go.

that thing that tries to stifle,
control, to frankly ruin your life,
i will tell you this in truth
—it lies.

this habit that used to help
you manage, numb or
somehow grasp control,
is no longer serving you at all

and you have suspected for
quite some time that you
are presently subservient
to it—instead.

addiction is a monstrous
taskmaster and if you do not
confront its favorite weapon,
denial, and throw heart and
soul into facing
your giant bold

that hurt, that experience,
the ogre that started
the pattern that you
were always desperately
trying to escape from . . .

then addiction
will likely win.

and i for one would
weep if this the case
becomes, for i have
seen this devastation
up close, to the person
—and to everyone they love.

i firmly believe you possess
intrinsic tools to support,
and a source of strength supreme
that has been submerged

forgotten, but is waiting
to rise to the surface to
enable you for such a
time as this.

and now is the time to rail
against all that lies,
to take your stand
and begin the fight for your life.
since this is exactly
what is at stake,
the battle to take back
the rest of your days.

do not be discouraged
if the path forward is one
that zigs and zags.
keep your goal
of freedom

in sight on the horizon
and the zigs will lessen
and the zags will only
your path correct
—just a little bit.

i believe
that you
can do this

your life will ring bright
and full and joyful
with the sound of healing
and freedom.

> — if you or anyone you care about is fighting
> addiction, then this is for you, with love.

I hope that you consider
that on this road that makes up life
you just might find hope
and inspiration
and purpose

and you might even experience
fulfilment in the end.

these things are possible
and everything like this that
you have ever longed for
can exist.

and today may be thick with
darkness but that does not
negate the reality
that there
is light.

   — there is always, always hope.

the egg shakes and then it cracks
as the chick inside fights its way
into the wide, wide world.

and while every parent wants
to ease the struggle, soften the
journey, lessen the blow

it is essential, the chick must
fight this battle for themselves.
for every great champion has

trained for the task and every
hero of legend has become strong
through the walk of life and the
lessons therein.

and everyone who does anything
of intrinsic value on this beautiful
ball of blue, is someone who has
discovered

that life isn't so much about
what you do, but is first and
most importantly about
the character
of who you are

and nothing can be gained by a chick
who has everything pried open
for them continual. this is the hope

that every parent must hold close
to their chest as they support
their offspring

while allowing them to learn
to succeed, and even to fail,
on their own.

perhaps this is the most difficult of
all lessons that a parent must
discover
—when to support
and when to let go.

i thought i had forgiven you
many trips around the sun ago
but today i discovered a niggle
a little pest folded within a thought.

because wherever you are in this
moment, i cannot wish you well
without a pause and
clenched teeth through a smile.

surprised by this notion disingenuous
i pause.

and discover that the wounds written
with your name once again need
a bit of gardening.

i am so deeply tired of this process
so truly disappointed that i must
once again think of you and prick
the sore so it can breathe.

i want this to be finished
but know the only way i can
truly be free, is to minister to
this pain, this anger
once again.

even though i will never forget,
the ripples are too wide and lasting

i can let go
choose to forgive

as many times as required
until my heart is at peace.

how can i explain to you
the dizzying disorientation
i feel

as we sit here in the present
talking about a topic that is
well and good

but for me it triggers and
takes me out of today into
times past

and my body, while perfectly
safe right now, remembers
a story different.

and even as my lips move,
i am breathing in deep and
slow

reminding myself
that i am here and now
and that i am secure

feeling the fabric of the sofa
beneath my fingers
and scanning the room.

even though this sounds
unpleasant, and it is,
i have dealt with it long.

and while this would have
had me reeling in the past,
feeling like my

body itself betrayed and would
send me to my bed shivering
for the day,

i am now more swiftly aware,
more armed with the thoughts
that will remind

that my body is my friend
and i appreciate its
attempts to protect

and whisper thanks
for its vigilance even though
in this moment fight, flight or freeze
is not required

and most of the time this relationship
with ptsd goes unnoticed now
by everyone
but me.

this place of sadness is not your home,
neither is the space that is anxiety.
you may visit them, yes, but your
true home is found in the place
of peace.

if peace is a bit dusty today
you can walk right in, broom in hand
the rightful owner of this house
and get to work

dusting off worries and surface cares
plumping the cushions, making the tea
and sitting down in front of fire friendly
to savor this place, this space, this peace
—your home.

peace can feel elusive, lost far off
in the distance, but is often just
a bit of intentionality and
sorting of self away.

while the storm may roar around
it does not need to rage within
since you, cognisant creation,
have the ability to sift through the
damage being done, evaluate,
shore up and reach out to all
you know that will bring
you peace, intentional.

so, take the time and space
to see, to act. you do not
have to just endure
the tempest.

as i sit beside and ponder
all the things that make up you,
the things you have done, your
accomplishments both small
and tremendous

it's the essence of who you
are that has mattered.

you have made a difference
to so many, going above and
beyond and always wearing
the face of the One whose
name you represent faithful

and i want to be more like you.
in fact, if i have heroes here upon
this earth, you are one of these

and now that your heart is tired
and your breathing will soon slow,
i find that in this i want to be like
you as well

for what will your eyes before long see
what faces will you encounter, what
sights will you behold?

and it will not be long until you hear
the words "well done" spoken loud
and long

and you can fold
into the arms of the One
who will never
let you go.

he sat, head hooded, sunglasses on
with the frame of someone you
might be careful walking past
on a darkened street at night.

but as he slouched over keys
at the piano by the supermarket,
he produced melodies both skilful
and tender, fully invested
in the nuances required to infuse
the song with meaning.

and i marveled at the courage
it took to express his soul
through music
for all around to enjoy
especially in this public place.

he gave a thumbs up but
tucked his head with shyness
when asked to play another.

and as you should never judge
a book by its cover, you should never
make assumptions about a
bulky-looking, hooded bloke.

(or anyone really for that matter)

their heart, it just might sing.

you hold out your hand
and say "come"

quiet and simple
the invitation ripples
through my mind

and i remember then
that while the waves
are high and the waters
deep, you are always
greater still

and while there are many
paths i have now tread,
i have not walked
a single step alone

and so once again i put
aside fear and doubt
and more than a bit of pride

while fully knowing and
accepting that
this will lead me beyond
my abilities alone

i step out on the water
and fix my eyes on the face
above the waves

after the winter,
you went for a walk in spring
and noticed signs of life
all around.

sparrows and seagulls and
even a flock of black swans
at the far end of the beach.

water sparkled and people
passed. trees bowed their
greetings and the breeze
felt like the start
of something new.

and your heart sighed deep
and long with the reminder
that you are too,
connected.

and the cobwebs that had
gathered in winter loosened
and melted away in sun.

try not to fall into traps of thinking
that leaning into
something that disturbs you
but you can do nothing about

and letting the 'upset' build
is actually *doing* something
to impact the problem.

it is not. it is simply robbing you
of peace that your soft
self is in desperate need
of wearing—and does absolutely
nothing to impart change

other than to change *you*
adding to stress, stealing
calm, thieving away
precious moments of life.

so what do you trust,
how do you make sense of good,
and where does your hope come from?

because the bigger your trust
the stronger your peace.
—this is where your true influence lies.

you tend to float away

        up

    up

up

into the atmosphere
like a helium balloon on string

not even noticing down below
what the body left behind
is doing.

lost in the clouds you drift, and
sometimes ponder deep and
thought provoking things, and

often you create. but sometimes it is
worry and cares and thoughts that
distract, dominate and eventually

distress. so in moments like these
you must shake your body awake,
reach up tippy-toes high
fingers stretched
to grab ahold of strings

and pull yourself gently back down
to earth with kindness and care
and then to offer yourself the solace

of this present moment, noticing all that is
miraculous within. because while beauty may be
observed from clouds, feet-on-earth grounded is

the space where all five senses engage and
this combined loveliness is absorbed,
perspective gained, breath upon breath.

the here-and-now, this moment, is where
balance is restored. and while later you might
begin to drift away again,

that tether will remain.

we are droplets
of water
clinging to leaves

who sometimes
feel we are only
barely holding on

but in the quiet rays
of early morning fresh,
we sparkle and gleam

even in those very first
beams of dawn and transform
into an element of beauty

glorious to all who pause
and take the moment to notice

—we simply required the light to shine

how did one small babe
fresh and soft and new

born in hope
swaddled in calm
alive in love

make the heavens
and angels sing
and hearts rejoice
down through the
ages?

he, the conduit
of peace, the expression
of how God himself
considers all of us.

this is grace
upon grace

and my wish for you
is that your soul
will feel its value
this day and
every day,

and that you will
never ever doubt
your worth again.

- breakup letter to anxiety -

i see you hiding over there
waiting, attempting to sneak
slowly into my day.

whispering already that there are
things beyond my control
to be considered.

dire things that, if only i would give
my time and energy to,
i *might* be able to solve

just by worrying a bit, or a lot.
this, the lie that you seek to
infuse into my brain.

but i have become steadily more aware
of your despicable ways
and you cannot come back in

willy-nilly any longer
for i despise
the things you do, to me
and to others around.

i have taken down the welcome sign,
brought in all the chairs.
we will no longer sip ice tea together
in the heat of midday or watch the sunset

—and especially will not commune
when night-time comes

stealing my sleep and flowing over
into dreams. no, you are not
welcome here anymore
or ever again
and i have initiated measures
to take back the life
you attempt to steal.

and while you might still
sneak up close from time to time
i see the signs that you are near
but you will never come to dine
or unpack your bag in my house again.

we are well and truly over and i hope
one day i will not even need to think or say your name.

my mind is set, notice has been given—so leave.

do you feel like you're in the waiting
hands outstretched but feet firmly planted?

heart thirsty for more, impatient
wrestling with restraints
that chafe.

and every day you wake
with expectation only to encounter
'stuck' once again.

this pause forced
does not of failure speak.

do you remember the bear
hibernating in den,
caterpillar cocooned,
bird resting upon nest?

it is nine long months before
a woman gives birth.

it may go against our grain
in this fast-paced place,
but there is always
an interval of wait.

and when we lash against that
which withholds, we only cause
more pain.

the season may be undesirable
unwanted
but there is always a purpose
for this
—so wait.

you feel ground up, crushed,
only a fragment of what you were.

and let's be honest, the process
has been painful.
but let me hearten you with this:

of crushed-up rock is metal made
and metal is vital in the formation
of concrete.

so instead of a life smashed apart
broken beyond repair,
you have been becoming the elements
of a foundation solid.

it might take some time.
you need to be further mixed,
processed
and shall require time to set

but what you become in the end
will weather any storm
solid.

yesterday while sitting
by the sea, a man jumped to his feet and
ran to shore, urgently gesticulating
—caution spread.

and then we saw the fin as well
not too close, but perhaps
not far enough away for comfort.

and observers rose
and swimmers emerged
and young ones gathered close . . .

until we saw
that instead of triangled,
the fin was curved

and in place of extreme caution,
delight ensued as creature
not everyday seen cavorted
in lazy afternoon sun.

and we pointed and *ahhh'd*
and as we later strolled away
i wondered

how much of life is spent
assuming a shark
when there is naught
but a dolphin instead?

when i came into this world
eyes wide and overwhelmed with wonder
i deduced that there was light here

and that the light was good
and what i wanted most in life
was to absorb as much of it as possible.

i desire this
with so much ferociousness
that i would give all i have
to grasp the coattails of light's last ray
even for a moment more to bask
in the glow.

perhaps this is what strengthens bones
when clouds cover sun
when the rains fall fierce
and darkness creeps ever nearer.

and if i have only one thing
to bequeath to you
it is this:

be a seeker, absorber and
passionate follower of the light
and then, by default
be a bearer of light to all
you meet.

so breathe in light until there is no
room for darkness left within your
frame. let light grip your hand and
never fear darkness again.

the clock ticks

-get-
    -on-
-your-
    -way-

there are jobs to be done, things to accomplish

but still
—pause
to take in the day
this momentary peace

remember to be present
look out the window
see the motion of the clouds
the soft movement of the palms
their fingerlike wave of 'hello' to the morn
with soft pink floss embracing the blues
the sky also wakes.

let your eyes wander, soak it all in
connect to the *now*, first.

remember who you are is not what you *do*.
you can do lots of things, but not really *be*.
if we focus on the step that's coming
we miss all of the *now*
then i wonder do we really even live?

this space, the foundation
the thing that carries you
your connection to the Source.

the hand still ticks, but now it speaks:

-stay-

      -present-

-be-

      -still-

      — take the pause, devotedly and often.

this is my humble apology
to all of the words that i didn't deem
'just right' to remain upon the page

that i heartlessly and callously
swept aside, deleted.

it wasn't that you weren't good enough,
your shape and form and personality
did please.

it was more about the general timing of
our meeting and your location upon the page.

so with that said, please know that honestly
it's not you

it's me, really . . .

and i genuinely hope
that we can
still.
be.
friends.

if you had told me way back then
through years of waiting long
i might not have believed

how high and low the rivers would flow
how frequent my steps would lead to joy
unbridled—but more often how they
would dance with pain.

in those days and months
heart bled and sorrow grew,
but then again
—so did love

she snuck in there like the first blooms
of spring, shimmering with dew—
every year a wonderment, unexpected.

you would think that pain would wither,
grind fragile hearts
to dust, but no . . .

love vocalised,
began to sing
full-throated and free

and with each breath grew
until at last i fell in love with all of it,
both the steps that sang and
those that wept.

the purpose of a journey is to end up
in a different and hopefully better
place than where you started . . .

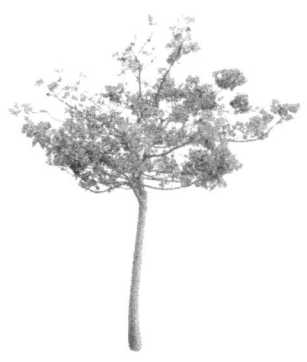

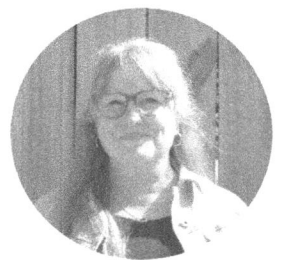

Heather Pound was born and raised in the USA but has lived more years outside of it now than in. Parts of her heart are in several other countries where she has spent time as well, but New Zealand, where she now lives with her husband, has become home. Heather has four adult children and one grandson. As a certified counsellor, she is a big fan of people in general and a great believer in the healing power of beauty. Themes of her work include mental well-being, humanity, nature, faith, relationships, motherhood and hope.

www.heatherpound.com

www.facebook.com/hlpound

@heatherpound